Projects

—

Every good life should be rich in projects: new approaches to how to get things done. Our projects might be for novels, businesses, film scripts, children, trips, home decoration schemes or political ambitions.

What unites all projects is that they need a safe initial place to germinate, somewhere with a lot of space and calm, where no one will laugh or ask the wrong sort of questions, and where first thoughts can carefully be built up into the robust proposals that the world will one day require of us.

A good project rarely comes to us in one go. Our minds tend to come up with fragments, which tumble out in the wrong order, at weird times of day and night. That's why we need a journal on hand to collect the fragments and allow us the opportunity to discern their logical shape and true identities. Working out what we really think and want is remarkably tricky. It might be the secret to a good life.

We're sometimes told that anyone can have a good idea, and that execution is all. This journal disagrees. Good ideas are very thin on the ground and easily get snuffed out. Giving up too soon is a constant danger. A project that a while back seemed full of promise (even a touch brilliant) can fade and succumb to a fatal lack of confidence, time or simple organisation.

Writing helps – as do diagrams, charts, lists, underlinings and spidery connecting arrows and pages of liberating crossings out. Our minds get in the mood at surprising moments. A thought falls into shape as you're boarding a plane; a new angle strikes you while waiting for a friend in a bar; stuck in traffic, a connection dawns on you and you feel compelled to reach for the journal before the lights change.

Our projects are a chance to externalise what's good inside us: things like creativity, rigour, wit, elegance – things developing in us that not everyone can see yet. A project is a statement of faith in the possibilities of our own growth.

To join The School of Life community and find out more,
scan below:

The School of Life publishes a range of books on essential topics in psychological and emotional life, including relationships, parenting, friendship, careers and fulfilment. The aim is always to help us to understand ourselves better and thereby to grow calmer, less confused and more purposeful. Discover our full range of titles, including books for children, here:

www.theschooloflife.com/books

The School of Life also offers a comprehensive therapy service, which complements, and draws upon, our published works:

www.theschooloflife.com/therapy